# MORNING FLEXIBILITY WORKOUTS

*7 minutes a day Low impact exercise for,Weight loss improved Joint movement, enhanced mobility, good posture and Core Strength*

Wayne K. Deck

# TABLE OF CONTENT

# INTRODUCTION

In the bustling metropolis of New Fountain lived a vibrant guy named Bruno, whose infectious energy was only equaled by his enthusiasm for life. Despite his zeal, Bruno was dealing with several health difficulties that appeared to be threatening his energy.

His employment required lengthy hours of sitting in front of a computer screen, resulting in knee stiffness and severe back pain. Bruno recognized the approaching dangers posed by his sedentary lifestyle, including the risk of tendinitis and bursitis, excess body weight, and increased weariness.

Bruno was determined to restore his health and well-being and sought a solution. In his search, he came upon a book named "Morning Flexibility Workouts," which proved to be the solution he needed. Bruno was intrigued by the book's potential to treat his bodily illnesses, so he quickly read its contents. Its precise exercises and routines provided a ray of hope amid his worries.

With renewed determination, Bruno began including morning flexibility training into his routine. What began as a simple promise quickly evolved into a transforming adventure. Bruno's general health and wellness improved dramatically as the days and weeks passed.

The stiffness in his knees eventually subsided, as did the constant backache. Energized by the positive changes he witnessed, Bruno embraced life with fresh enthusiasm and vitality. Bruno overcame his physical obstacles and gained a new understanding of the importance of proactive self-care. With each stretch and bend, he fostered both his body and his spirit, cultivating a sense of balance and harmony inside himself. Bruno's journey to optimal health demonstrated the transforming potential of embracing change and prioritizing one's well-being.

# CHAPTER ONE

## *Benefits of Morning Flexibility Workouts*

Morning flexibility activities provide numerous benefits that can greatly improve your general fitness and well-being. First and foremost, doing flexibility exercises in the morning wakes up your body and prepares it for the day ahead. Gently stretching your muscles and joints increases blood flow and circulation, which can boost your energy and mental alertness throughout the day.

Early flexibility training might help you improve your posture and lower your chance of injury while exercising or going about your daily routine. Stretching and elongating your muscles daily can help to correct imbalances and relieve tightness, resulting in improved alignment and less pressure on the body.

Another significant advantage of early flexibility training is its potential to promote calm and stress reduction. Beginning the day with moderate stretching and deep breathing exercises can help to quiet your mind and reduce muscle tension, leaving you feeling more relaxed and focused as you face the day's difficulties.

Incorporating flexibility exercises into your morning routine can help you gain flexibility and range of motion over time. This enhanced flexibility not only allows you to move more easily and comfortably throughout the day but also lowers your risk of muscle stiffness and joint pain, particularly as you get older.

In addition to the physical benefits, morning flexibility training can improve your emotional health. establishing aside time each morning to focus on yourself and your well-being can improve your attitude and self-esteem, establishing a good tone for the remainder of the day.

Generally, including early flexibility activities in your daily regimen can improve your physical health, mental well-being, and general quality of life. Whether you want to boost your energy, reduce stress, or improve your flexibility, beginning your day with a few simple stretches can make a big difference.

## *Setting Realistic Goals*

Setting realistic goals is critical for success in your fitness journey, especially when including early flexibility routines. First, evaluate your present level of flexibility and establish specific, measurable, attainable, relevant, and time-bound (SMART) objectives.

For example, if you can't touch your toes, set a goal of improving hamstring and lower back flexibility within a specific time frame, such as being able to touch your toes comfortably in three months.

When setting goals, think about your lifestyle and schedule. If you only have a few minutes in the morning, begin with five to ten-minute flexibility programs that target specific muscle groups. Gradually increase the duration and intensity of your workouts as your flexibility grows. Always listen to your body and don't push yourself too hard, especially if you're new to fitness or have previous injuries.

Divide your larger flexibility goals into smaller milestones. Celebrate each milestone along the way, whether it's achieving a new range of motion or holding a stretch for a longer time. These modest triumphs will keep you motivated and strengthen your dedication to your fitness goals.

Maintain flexibility with your goals as your body changes and grows. Be willing to change your timeframe or training program based on your changing demands and priorities. If you have setbacks, such as tightness or soreness, reassess your approach and make any required changes to avoid injury and preserve consistency.

Maintain accountability and motivation by tracking your progress regularly. Keep a workout journal or utilize fitness monitoring apps to track your flexibility progress and reflect on your accomplishments. Celebrate your accomplishments and learn from any setbacks you face along the way. Setting realistic goals and sticking to your morning flexibility routines will improve your general health and well-being in the long run.

## *Importance of Consistency*

Consistency in early flexibility training is essential for attaining the best results and maintaining overall health and wellness. When you stick to a consistent regimen, you train your body to adapt and improve over time. Here's why consistency is important:

***Progression:*** Consistently performing morning flexibility exercises allows your body to progress and improve flexibility over time. Regular stretching gradually increases your range of motion and reduces muscular stiffness, resulting in increased flexibility.

***Injury Prevention:*** Regular flexibility exercises help to maintain the elasticity of your muscles, tendons, and ligaments. This lowers the risk of injury during physical activities throughout the day by encouraging better movement mechanics and joint stability.

***Muscle Recovery:*** Consistent morning flexibility workouts help the recovery process by increasing blood flow to the muscles and tissues. This reduces discomfort, stiffness, and tension, allowing your body to recover faster and perform better in future sessions.

***Mental Clarity:*** Beginning your day with a consistent morning flexibility program can also provide mental advantages. It helps to clear your mind, increase attention, and reduce tension, creating a good tone for the day.

***Habit Formation:*** Consistency creates habits. Establishing a consistent morning flexibility routine creates a habit that becomes imprinted in your everyday life. This makes it easier to stay on your fitness plan in the long run, resulting in sustained progress and general health.

Consistency in morning flexibility workouts is critical for increasing flexibility, reducing injuries, facilitating muscle recovery, improving mental clarity, and developing long-term habits for a healthier lifestyle. Maintain your routine, and you will enjoy physical and emotional rewards.

## *Safety Precautions*

To avoid injury during early flexibility training, prioritize safety precautions. Warm up for 5-10 minutes with modest cardiovascular workouts, such as jogging or jumping jacks, to boost blood flow to your muscles. Following that, do dynamic stretches like arm circles and leg swings to gradually loosen joints and improve flexibility.

Maintain good form throughout the exercise to avoid strain or overexertion. Listen to your body and don't push beyond discomfort into pain. Progress gently, increasing intensity or length only when you are ready and comfortable with your present level of activity.

Stay hydrated before, during, and after your workout to ensure proper muscle function and avoid dehydration. Dress appropriately for the weather and use breathable, moisture-wicking textiles to keep comfortable during exercise.

Invest in supportive footwear for stability and cushioning, especially if your workouts include jumping or impact. Consider using yoga mats or resistance bands to improve your workout experience while lowering your chance of sliding or injury.

Don't skip the cooling exercises. Spend 5-10 minutes doing static stretches to gradually lower your heart rate and enhance muscle recovery. Pay attention to any indicators of discomfort or pain and alter your routine as needed to achieve a safe and effective morning flexibility workout.

# *How to Use This Book*

Set your goals. Before getting in, determine your flexibility goals. Do you want to increase general flexibility, focus on specific muscle groups, or improve mobility for a specific sport or activity?

***Understand Your Body:*** Identify your present level of flexibility, as well as any areas of tightness or discomfort. This allows you to personalize the workouts to your specific needs.

Begin slowly with easy stretches to warm up your muscles and prepare for more strenuous flexibility exercises. To ease into the regimen, practice deep breathing and relaxation.

***Follow the Structure:*** This book is designed to gradually increase the intensity and intricacy of the stretches. Begin with the basic workouts and proceed to more advanced routines as you gain strength and flexibility.

***Listen to your body:*** Pay attention to how your body reacts to each stretch. Avoid pushing yourself too hard and risking damage. Modify workouts to meet any limits or discomfort.

***Be Consistent:*** Set aside time each morning to do your flexibility routine. Consistency is essential for long-term improvement.

***Track Your Progress:*** This book has a workout Planner to document your flexibility goals, accomplishments, and any difficulties you have along the road. This will help you stay motivated and monitor your development over time.

***Stay Hydrated and Nourished:*** Proper hydration and nutrition are critical for maintaining flexibility and general health. Drink plenty of water and eat nutrient-dense foods to improve your performance.

***Seek practitioner Advice:*** If you have any pre-existing medical ailments or concerns, speak with a healthcare practitioner or experienced fitness trainer before beginning a new flexibility routine.

Enjoy the process. Embrace the process of increasing your flexibility and mobility. Celebrate your accomplishments and stay focused on your health and wellness goals.

## *Equipment Needed*

Morning flexibility workouts require minimum equipment to maximize your routine. Begin with a yoga mat to provide comfort and stability during floor activities. Choose a mat with enough thickness to cushion your joints. Next, consider using resistance bands of varied strengths to increase resistance and deepen stretches.

These bands are adaptable, allowing them to effectively target certain muscle groups. A foam roller is also useful for self-myofascial release, which promotes muscle repair and increases flexibility. Choose a foam roller with a reasonable density to apply enough pressure without causing discomfort.

A stability ball is another effective tool for improving flexibility and balance. Use it for core-strengthening activities and to test stability during stretches.

Also use  basic towel or strap to help deepen stretches and improve flexibility, especially in hard-to-reach places like the shoulders and hamstrings.

Consider using a yoga block to adjust poses and accommodate different levels of flexibility. It can provide support and stability, allowing you to comfortably try out deeper stretches.

With these key pieces of equipment, you may easily engage in morning flexibility workouts, which promote mobility, avoid injury, and improve general well-being. Start your day off right by focusing on flexibility and mobility with these multipurpose tools.

# CHAPTER TWO

## Warm-up Routine

A solid warm-up routine is necessary before beginning your morning flexibility training. Begin with dynamic stretching exercises to promote blood flow and get your muscles ready for movement. To progressively release your joints and muscles, try exercises like arm circles, leg swings, and torso twists.

Next, integrate dynamic motions that replicate the workouts you'll be performing during your workout. For example, if you want to undertake yoga postures or leg stretches, incorporate dynamic lunges or high knees to engage the muscles you will be using.

After active stretching, switch to static stretches to increase flexibility. Stretch major muscular groups, such as the hamstrings, quadriceps, calves, and back. Hold each stretch for 15-30 seconds, making sure you feel a soft pull without any pain.

Pay attention to your breathing while you warm up. Inhale deeply through your nose and exhale gently through your mouth to oxygenate your muscles and relax your nervous system.

As you go through your warm-up routine, progressively increase the intensity of your motions while keeping good form. Listen to your body and alter your range of motion as needed to avoid overstretching or straining muscles.

Include balance exercises such as single-leg stands or tree poses in your workout to improve stability and prevent injury.

Stay hydrated and energize your body with a light snack or pre-exercise meal before your morning workout.

## *Dynamic Stretching*

Dynamic stretching is a type of stretching that requires continuous movement over the entire range of motion. It contrasts with static stretching, which involves holding a stretch for an extended length of time. Dynamic stretching is useful for morning flexibility workouts because it increases blood flow to muscles and joints, enhancing range of motion and lowering the chance of injury.

When conducting dynamic stretching in the morning, select activities that target the key muscle groups you'll use throughout the day. This comprises leg swings, arm circles, hip circles, and torso twists. These exercises serve to warm up the muscles and get them ready for activities.

During your morning flexibility program, concentrate on making each dynamic stretch smooth and rhythmic. Avoid jumping or jerking motions, as they can result in damage. Instead, progress through each exercise carefully, increasing the range of motion as your muscles release.

Dynamic stretching can be customized to meet your individual needs and fitness level. Begin with easier exercises and move to more difficult ones as your flexibility improves.

Including dynamic stretching in your morning routine can provide multiple benefits, including increased flexibility, better athletic performance, and a lower chance of injury. Make it a regular component of your morning fitness routine to receive the most benefits.

# *Joint Mobilization Exercises*

Joint Mobilization Exercise is vital for increasing flexibility and mobility, especially in the morning when your body may be tight after sleep. These exercises include gently moving your joints through their whole range of motion to lubricate them and stimulate blood flow, which helps to relieve stiffness and reduces the chance of injury throughout the day.

Begin your morning flexibility regimen with dynamic stretches like arm circles, leg swings, and torso twists to warm up your muscles and prepare them for action. Then, focus on joint mobility exercises that target particular regions such as the neck, shoulders, spine, hips, knees, and ankles.

To relax the cervical spine, gently move your head from side to side, nodding up and down and leaning your ear toward your shoulder. Next, enhance upper-body mobility with shoulder circles, arm swings, and wrist circles.

Moving down the spine, use movements like cat-cow stretches, spinal twists, and pelvic tilts to increase flexibility and reduce back strain. Hip circles, leg swings, and hip flexor stretches can all help you expand your range of motion and mobility.

Attention should be given to the lower-body joints. Knee circles, ankle circles, and toe touches can help to release the knees, ankles, and feet. To avoid injury, practice smooth, controlled motions and avoid pushing any joint beyond its natural range of motion.

Incorporate these joint mobilization exercises into your morning flexibility regimen to begin the day feeling limber, energized, and ready to face whatever obstacles come your way. Remember to listen to your body and adjust the exercises as needed to accommodate your specific flexibility and mobility levels. Consistent practice will result in considerable

improvements in your total joint health and
flexibility over time.

## *Cardiovascular Warm-up*

When beginning your morning flexibility workout, start with a cardiovascular warm-up to prepare your body for the activities ahead. A cardiovascular warm-up is doing low- to moderate-intensity activities that raise your heart rate and boost blood flow to the muscles.

Begin your warm-up with 5-10 minutes of vigorous motions like running in place, jumping jacks, or high knees. These activities progressively increase your heart rate and body temperature, preparing your muscles and joints for the upcoming stretching and flexibility exercises.

Incorporate exercises that imitate the actions you'll be doing during your workout to target the appropriate muscles and joints. For example, if your flexibility practice involves leg stretches, add vigorous leg swings or lunges to your warm-up.

During your warm-up, focus on appropriate form and technique to avoid injury and get the most out of your workout. Pay attention to your breathing and try to keep a consistent rhythm during your warm-up.

As you proceed through your warm-up, progressively increase the intensity of your motions to raise your heart rate and prepare your body for more strenuous activity. To minimize weariness or overexertion, don't push yourself too hard during the warm-up.

After you've finished your cardiovascular warm-up, ease into your flexibility exercises, making sure to stretch each major muscle group properly. A correct warm-up in your morning flexibility routine prepares you for a safe and productive workout, allowing you to develop your flexibility, avoid injury, and maximize your performance.

## *Importance of Warm-up*

When beginning your morning flexibility workout, start with a cardiovascular warm-up to prepare your body for the activities ahead. A cardiovascular warm-up is doing low- to moderate-intensity activities that raise your heart rate and boost blood flow to the muscles.

Begin your warm-up with 5-10 minutes of vigorous motions like running in place, jumping jacks, or high knees. These activities progressively increase your heart rate and body temperature, preparing your muscles and joints for the upcoming stretching and flexibility exercises.

Incorporate exercises that imitate the actions you'll be doing during your workout to target the appropriate muscles and joints. For example, if your flexibility practice involves leg stretches, add vigorous leg swings or lunges to your warm-up.

During your warm-up, focus on appropriate form and technique to avoid injury and get the most out of your workout. Pay attention to your breathing and try to keep a consistent rhythm during your warm-up.

As you proceed through your warm-up, progressively increase the intensity of your motions to raise your heart rate and prepare your body for more strenuous activity. To minimize weariness or overexertion, don't push yourself too hard during the warm-up.

After you've finished your cardiovascular warm-up, ease into your flexibility exercises, making sure to stretch each major muscle group properly. A correct warm-up in your morning flexibility routine prepares you for a safe and productive workout, allowing you to develop your flexibility, avoid injury, and maximize your performance.

## Sample Warm-up Routines

When it comes to morning flexibility workouts, it's critical to start the day with a regimen that not only prepares your body for activity but also increases your flexibility. Here's a whole warm-up program designed just for mornings:

***Dynamic Stretching (5-10 minutes):*** Start with dynamic stretches to wake up your muscles and boost blood flow. Make leg swings, arm circles, torso twists, and shoulder rolls. These motions work for numerous muscle groups and increase flexibility.

***Joint Mobilization (3-5 minutes):*** Work on mobilizing your joints to increase their range of motion. Make mild motions like neck circles, wrist circles, ankle rotations, and hip circles. This relieves stiffness and prepares your joints for more strenuous action.

***Sun Salutations (5-10 minutes):*** Use yoga-inspired sun salutations to increase flexibility and relaxation. Flow through a series of postures, including mountain pose, forward fold, plank, cobra pose, and downward-facing dog. Coordination of breath with each action has a relaxing impact on both the mind and the body.

***Foam rolling (3-5 minutes):*** Use a foam roller to relax stiff muscles. Focus on the calves, hamstrings, quadriceps, glutes, and back. Roll slowly and halt in any sensitive areas to enable the muscle to relax.

***Dynamic Movements (5-7 minutes):*** Practice dynamic movements that correspond to the tasks you'll be undertaking later in your exercise or everyday routine. Include movements such as leg swings, arm circles, high knees, and buttock kicks. This improves coordination and prepares the body for certain motions.

Breathing Exercises (2-3 minutes): To finish your warm-up, do deep breathing exercises to concentrate your mind and oxygenate your body. Sit or stand tall, inhale deeply through your nose to expand your diaphragm, and expel completely through your mouth. Repeat multiple breath cycles.

Listen to your body and adjust the intensity of each workout accordingly. Consistency is essential, so work this morning flexibility exercise into your daily calendar to gain the full advantages of increased flexibility and general well-being.

# *Tips for Effective Warm-ups*

***Start gradually:*** Begin your warm-up with easy activities that gradually raise your heart rate and warm your muscles. This might be mild running in place or quick walking.

***Dynamic Stretches:*** Use dynamic stretches to simulate the movements you'll be doing during your exercise. Leg swings, arm circles, and hip rotations can all help you enhance your flexibility and range of motion.

Warm up with a focus on main muscular areas such as the legs, back, chest, and shoulders. Perform dynamic stretches and motions that target these areas to prepare them for the next workout.

***Joint Mobility Exercises:*** Include exercises that improve joint mobility and flexibility, such as wrist circles, ankle rolls, and neck rotations. This helps to lubricate the joints and relieves stiffness.

***Progressive Warm-up:*** Gradually increase the intensity of your warm-up as you proceed. Begin with milder motions and progressively raise the intensity to get your body ready for more strenuous exercise.

Concentrate on deep, regular breathing during your warm-up. This helps to oxygenate your muscles and prepares you mentally for the next activity.

***keep Hydrated:*** Drink water before, during, and after your warm-up to keep hydrated and perform optimally.

***Listen to your body:*** Pay attention to your body's sensations throughout the warm-up. If you feel any pain or discomfort, alter the workouts or check with a fitness specialist.

Balance activities, such as single-leg stands or yoga positions, can help to enhance stability and proprioception.

***Transition seamlessly:*** Once you've finished your warm-up, seamlessly transition into your primary workout, keeping the momentum and energy you've gained.

# *CHAPTER THREE*

## *Flexibility Exercises for Upper Body*

Start softly turning your neck clockwise and counterclockwise. To loosen up the neck muscles, perform 10-15 rotations in each direction.

***Shoulder Rolls:*** Stand tall and move your shoulders backward in a circular motion, then reverse. Perform 10-15 rolls in each direction to improve shoulder flexibility.

***Arm Circles:*** Extend your arms to the sides and form tiny circles, gradually increasing in size. Perform 10-15 circles forward and backward to improve shoulder and arm flexibility.

***Triceps Stretch:*** Raise one arm above and bend it, then extend your hand to the opposite shoulder blade. Using your other hand, gently press the elbow further. Hold for 15-30 seconds then swap sides.

***Chest Opener:*** Interlace your fingers behind your back, straighten your arms, and raise them slightly while pushing your shoulder blades together. Hold for 15–30 seconds to stretch the chest muscles.

***Upper Back Stretch:*** Sit or stand tall, clasp your hands in front of you, and round your upper back by pushing your hands out from your body. Hold for 15–30 seconds to stretch the upper back.

***Shoulder Stretch:*** Bring one arm across your body at shoulder height, then gently bring the other hand closer to your chest. Hold for 15-30 seconds then swap sides.

***Upper Body Twist:*** Sit or stand up straight, stretch your arms to the sides, and twist your body to one side while gazing over your shoulder. repeat on the opposite side after holding for Hold for 15-30 seconds

*Wrist Flexibility:* Extend one arm in front of you, palm down, and slowly draw the fingers back with the other hand to extend the wrist. Hold for 15-30 seconds then swap sides.

*Backbend Stretch:* Stand with your feet hip-width apart, hands on your lower back, and gradually arch backward while gazing up at the ceiling. Hold for 15–30 seconds to extend the chest and back.

Performing these flexibility exercises in the morning wakes up your muscles, increases circulation, and sets a good tone for the day.

Take deep breaths and listen to your body, avoiding painful movements. Consistency is crucial, so include these workouts in your regular regimen for the best results.

## *Neck Stretches*

When including neck stretches into your daily flexibility routines, it is critical to do it appropriately to minimize injury and optimize their benefits. Begin by sitting or standing tall with your shoulders relaxed and your spine in neutral alignment. This is a complete guide to effective neck stretches.

***Neck Rotation:*** Gently move your head to one side until you feel a comfortable stretch along the side of your neck.

Hold for 15-30 seconds, then switch to the opposite side.

Repeat 2-3 times per side.

***Neck Tilt:*** Slowly tilt your head to one side, placing your ear near your shoulder.

On the other side of you neck a stretch Should be felt on

Hold for 15-30 seconds, then swap sides. Repeat 2-3 times per side.

***Neck Flexion and Extension:*** Lower your chin to your chest and feel a stretch on the back of your neck.

Hold for 15-30 seconds, then gently tilt your head back to stare at the ceiling.

Across the front of your neck, a stretch should be felt.

Hold for 15–30 seconds.

For the next two or three times the procedure should be repeated.

***Shoulder Shrugs:*** Lift your shoulders to your ears and hold them for a few seconds before relaxing them.

Repeat the action 5-10 times to relieve tension in your neck and shoulders.

***Chin Tucks:*** Sit or stand tall and softly tuck your chin into your chest, forming a double chin.

Release after holding for 5-10 seconds

Repeat 5-10 times to strengthen the muscles in the front of your neck and improve posture.

***Ear-to- Shoulder strain:*** Slowly bring one ear to your shoulder, feeling a strain on the side of your neck.
Hold for 15-30 seconds and then swap sides. Repeat 2-3 times per side.

Always take slow breaths and never force a stretch beyond your comfort level. Incorporating these neck exercises into your morning practice can help you increase flexibility, reduce stiffness, and maintain general neck health. If you have any worries or already have neck

difficulties, listen to your body and check with a
fitness specialist.

## *Shoulder Mobility Drills*

To enhance shoulder mobility, include a range of drills in your morning flexibility routines. Begin with dynamic stretches such as arm circles, rotating your arms forward and backward to warm up the shoulder joints. Next, execute shoulder dislocations with a resistance band or a broomstick, progressively extending your grasp to improve flexibility.

Follow up with workouts that target particular muscle groups. For the rotator cuff, use a resistance band or light dumbbells to do internal and external rotations. These exercises strengthen the muscles around the shoulder joint, increasing stability and mobility.

Stretches like the cross-body shoulder stretch and the overhead triceps stretch can help you enhance your range of motion. Hold each stretch for 15-30 seconds, concentrating on muscular relaxation and deep breathing.

Incorporate mobility drills, such as the wall slide exercise, which involves pressing your arms against a wall and sliding them overhead while maintaining your back flat. This improves shoulder mobility while working the muscles of the upper back.

Don't forget to consider mobility in several planes of movement. Include exercises such as the shoulder YWT stretch, which improves shoulder mobility in several directions. Perform each action carefully and with control, emphasizing quality over quantity.

Finish your exercise with self-myofascial release, which uses a foam roller or lacrosse ball to relieve tension in the muscles surrounding the shoulder joint. Spend more time on regions that are tight or sore.

Consistency and appropriate technique are critical for improving shoulder mobility. By implementing these activities into your morning routine, you'll progressively improve flexibility,

lower your chance of injury, and improve overall
shoulder health.

## *Chest Opener*



Including chest openers in your morning flexibility training regimen is an excellent way to get your day started correctly. These exercises focus on the chest muscles, shoulders, and upper back, helping to offset the consequences of slouching and sitting for long durations.

To begin, perform a basic standing chest stretch. Stand tall, feet hip-width apart, and hands clasped behind your back.

Straighten your arms and gradually raise them away from your body, experiencing a stretch in your chest and shoulders.

Hold this posture for 20-30 seconds, taking deep breaths. Next, perform a doorway stretch.

With elbows bent at a 90-degree angle and forearms resting against the door frame Stand in a doorway

Step forward on one foot, letting your chest expand as you lean into the stretch. Hold for 20-30 seconds and then swap legs.

The Cobra yoga stance is another great way to expand your chest. Lie face down on the floor, with your hands squarely below your shoulders.

Lift your chest off the ground, pressing into your palms while maintaining your hips and knees firmly on the ground.

Hold for 20-30 seconds, concentrating on extending from the front of your body.

The Eagle Arms position provides a deeper stretch. Sit or stand tall, then cross your right arm beneath your left, wrapping your forearms around each other.

Raise your elbows to shoulder height and push your palms together. Lift your elbows slightly as you widen your chest and feel a stretch between your shoulder blades. Hold for 20-30 seconds and then swap sides.

Incorporate these chest openers into your morning flexibility exercise to improve posture, reduce stress, and increase mobility.

Ensure to breathe deeply and listen to your body, gradually increasing the intensity of the stretches as you gain comfort.

Begin your day feeling invigorated, open, and prepared to face whatever comes your way!

# *Arm and Wrist Stretches*

Morning flexibility routines are essential for getting your body ready for the day ahead, and concentrating on arm and wrist stretches may improve your general flexibility and mobility. Begin by standing tall, feet hip-width apart, and arms relaxed at your sides.

***Wrist Flexor Stretch:*** Extend your right arm in front of you, palm down.

With your left hand, gently press your right hand downward until you feel a stretch down the bottom of your forearm.

Swap side's after holding for 15 - 30 seconds

***Wrist Extensor Stretch:*** Hold your right arm out in front of you, palm up.

With your left hand, gently press your right hand backward until you feel a stretch at the top of your forearm.

Swap side's after holding for 15 - 30 seconds

***Triceps Stretch:*** Raise your right arm above and bend it till your right-hand touches the center of your back.

With your left hand, gently push your right elbow toward your head until you feel a stretch down the back of your arm.

Swap side's after holding for 15 - 30 seconds

***Bicep Stretch:*** Extend your right arm to the side, parallel to the floor, palm up.

With your right hand behind your head,Bend your elbow

Using your left hand, gently press your right elbow backward until you feel a stretch across the front of your arm.

Swap side's after holding for 15 - 30 seconds

***Forearm Stretch:*** Extend your right arm in front of you, palm down.

Using your left hand, gently press your right fingers back towards your body until you feel a stretch down your forearm.

Swap side's after holding for 15 - 30 seconds.

Including these arm and wrist stretches in your morning flexibility practice can help boost blood flow to these regions, reduce stiffness, and enhance range of motion, setting a good tone for the day. To avoid damage, always breathe deeply and never push yourself beyond your comfort level during stretching.

# Upper Back and Spine Stretching

Morning flexibility routines should include extending your upper back and spine to maintain excellent posture, reduce tension, and avoid injuries. Here's a detailed guide to assist you in successfully extending these areas:

**Cat-Cow Stretch:** Beggin on your hands and knees, placing your wrists precisely under your shoulders and your knees beneath your hips.

Inhale as you arch your back, lowering your belly to the floor and raising your head and tailbone to the ceiling (Cow).

Exhale while rounding your back, lowering your chin to your chest, and drawing your belly button against your spine (Cat). Repeat this flow for 8-10 repetitions.

**Child's Pose:** Sit back on your heels and extend your arms forward, dropping your chest to the floor and maintaining your hips above your heels. Place your forehead on the ground and relax into the stretch, feeling a slight extension of your spine and upper back.

focusing on deep breathing, hold for the next 30 - 60 seconds

**Thoracic Extension:** Sit on the floor, knees bent, feet flat on the ground. Position a foam roller horizontally behind your mid back.

Support your head with your hands as you slowly lean back over the roller, letting it gradually stretch your upper back.

Keep your hips down and avoid arching your lower back. Hold for 20-30 seconds and repeat as necessary.

**Thread the Needle:** Start on your hands and knees, then reach your right arm under your left arm and thread the needle through until your shoulder and temple are resting on the ground. Keep your left hand on the floor for support and hold the stretch for 20-30 seconds. Repeat on the opposite side.

***Upper Back and Shoulder Stretch:*** Stand tall with your feet hip-width apart. Clasp your hands in front of you and extend your arms.

Slowly raise your arms upward while maintaining them straight, until you feel a stretch in your upper back and shoulders. Hold for 20-30 seconds and then release.

Include these exercises in your morning routine to increase flexibility, reduce stiffness, and support general spine health. Listen to your body and stretch within your acceptable range of motion to avoid strain or damage. To achieve the best benefits, execute these stretches regularly.

## *Stretching Routine for the Upper Body*

A daily upper-body stretching regimen is essential for starting the day with maximum flexibility. Begin by concentrating on dynamic stretches to wake up your muscles and improve blood flow. Arm circles, shoulder rolls, and neck rotations will gently mobilize your joints and warm up your upper body.

Next, perform static stretches to lengthen and relax your muscles. Begin with a chest stretch, clasping your hands behind your back and slowly lifting your arms up to open your chest. Hold for 15-30 seconds, inhaling deeply.

Perform a triceps stretch by raising one arm above and bending it, with your hand behind your neck. With your other hand, gently press your elbow toward the middle of your back.

On each side Hold for 15–30 seconds

Next, extend your shoulders by bringing one arm across your body and pressing it on your chest with the opposing hand. Hold for 15-30 seconds then swap sides.

Continue with a back stretch by sitting on the floor with your legs outstretched. Reach your arms as far forward as possible, experiencing a slight stretch in your back and shoulders. Hold for 15-30 seconds, inhaling deeply.

To extend your neck muscles. Gently tilt your head to one side, moving your ear closer to your shoulder, until you feel a stretch on the other side of your neck. Hold for 15-30 seconds then swap sides.

Perform each stretch carefully and without bouncing, which might result in harm. To improve relaxation and flexibility, practice deep breathing throughout the workout. Incorporating this full upper-body stretching technique into your morning workout routine will not only improve your flexibility but will also establish a good tone for the rest of the day.

# CHAPTER FOUR

## *Flexibility Exercises for Lower Body*

Morning flexibility activities for your lower body are essential for maintaining general mobility and avoiding injuries during the workday. Here's a comprehensive guide to excellent flexibility exercises.

**Dynamic Warm-Up:** Start with dynamic motions to promote blood flow and relax your muscles.

Leg swings, leg circles, and hip circles are all exercises that target the lower body.

To stretch your hamstrings, sit on the floor with one leg extended and the other bowed. while keeping your back straight, reach towards your toes

Hold for 15-30 seconds then swap legs. Repeat 2–3 times.

***Quadriceps Stretch:*** Stand tall and grasp one foot behind you with your hand. Gently lift your foot towards your glutes, keeping your knees together. Hold for 15-30 seconds then swap sides. Repeat 2–3 times.

***Calf Stretch:*** Stand facing a wall, one foot in front of the other. Lean forward with your rear leg straight and heel on the ground. Hold for 15-30 seconds then swap sides. Repeat 2–3 times.

***Hip Flexor Stretch:*** Form a 90-degree angle by kneeling on one knee and bringing the other foot in front of you.

Lean forward and extend the front of your hip.

Hold for 15-30 seconds then swap sides.
Repeat 2–3 times.

Sit on the floor with your feet together and your knees bent to the sides.

Gently press your knees to the floor using your elbows

Hold for 15-30 seconds, then repeat 2-3 times.

***Glute Stretch:*** Lie on your back, one ankle crossed over the opposing knee.

Until you feel a stretch in the glutes,Pull the uncrossed leg towards your chest

Hold for 15-30 seconds then swap sides. Repeat 2–3 times.

***Foam Rolling:*** Finish your morning routine with foam rolling to relieve any leftover muscular tension. Concentrate on the hamstrings, quadriceps, calves, and glutes.

Add these flexibility exercises into your morning routine to increase lower-body mobility, boost performance, and lessen your risk of injury throughout the day. To get the most out of each stretch, execute it gently and hold it for an appropriate amount of time. Maintain consistency, and you will see gains in your flexibility over time.

# Hip Flexor Stretches

***Kneeling Hip Flexor Stretch:*** Start in a kneeling position with one foot front, knee bent at a 90-degree angle. Gently lean forward while maintaining your back straight, and push your hips forward. Swap legs after holding for 20-30 seconds

***Pigeon Pose:*** Start in a plank position, then raise one knee forward between your hands. Lower your body, preferably resting on your forearms. You should get a deep stretch in the hip of the outstretched leg. Hold for 20 to 30 seconds before swapping sides.

***Standing Hip Flexor Stretch:*** Stand tall and place one foot slightly in front of the other. Engage your core and gradually tilt your pelvis backward, forcing your hips forward. Swap legs after holding for 20-30 seconds

Supine Hip Flexor Stretch: Lie on your back, knees bent, feet flat on the floor. Bring one knee to your chest and grip behind the thigh.

Slowly stretch the opposite leg straight out to the floor. You should feel a stretch in the front hip of the outstretched leg.  Swap legs after holding for 20-30 seconds

**Bridge Pose:** Lie on your back, knees bent and feet flat on the floor, hip width apart. Lift your hips to the ceiling, tightening your glutes and activating your core. Before lowering back down,Hold for a few seconds

**Low Lunge with Side Bend:** Begin in a low lunge, one leg on the ground and the other foot ahead. Reach both arms aloft and bend gently to the side to feel a stretch along the rear leg's hip flexor. Hold for 20-30 seconds then swap sides.

**Frog Stretch:** Start on all fours and gradually expand your knees apart, maintaining your ankles in line with your knees. Lower your hips to the ground and rest your forearms. Hold for 20-30 seconds to feel a deep stretch in the inner thighs and hip flexors.

***Seated Butterfly Stretch:*** Sit on the floor, soles of your feet together, knees bent out to the sides. While sitting upright, hold onto your feet and gently press your knees to the floor. Hold for 20-30 seconds, experiencing the stretch in your inner thighs and hip flexors.

***Seated Spinal Twist:*** Sit on the floor, legs outstretched in front of you. Bend one knee and cross it over the opposing leg, with the foot flat on the floor. Twist your body towards the bent knee and gently press your opposing elbow into the outside of the knee. Hold for 20-30 seconds then swap sides.

***Happy Baby Pose:*** Lie on your back, bringing both knees to your chest. Grab the outside borders of your feet with your hands, then slowly draw your knees towards the floor beside your torso. Hold for 20-30 seconds, feeling the stretch in your hips and groin.

Including these exercises throughout your morning routine to boost flexibility, mobility, and hip health. Always take deep breaths and pay attention to your body's indications when stretching.

# *Hamstring Stretching*

The Standing Forward Bend, also known as Uttanasana in yoga, is a position in which you fold forward from the hips while standing and bring your hands toward or to the ground. It is great for extending the hamstrings, calves, and hips, as well as relaxing the mind and alleviating tension.

The Seated Forward Fold, or Paschimottanasana in yoga, includes. sitting on the floor with extended legs and folding forward from the hips, reaching for the feet or beyond while maintaining the spine straight. It's fantastic for extending the spine, hamstrings, and lower back, as well as relaxing the mind and boosting digestion.

***Standing Towel Stretch:***
The Standing Towel Stretch is a flexibility exercise that involves holding a towel behind your back with both hands and gently pulling one hand up while pulling the other down,

extending the shoulders and chest muscles. It is useful for increasing shoulder flexibility and alleviating stress in the upper body.

### Seated single-leg hamstring stretch:

The sitting single-leg hamstring stretch is an excellent method for stretching your hamstring muscles. Sit on the floor, one leg stretched straight in front of you and the other bent, with the foot on the extended leg's inner thigh.

 Lean forward from your hips while maintaining your back straight, then reach for your toes until you feel a stretch at the back of your extended leg. Switch legs after holding the stretch for 15-30 seconds,Repeat as required.

### Lying Hamstring Stretch:

Lie on your back, legs straight.

One of your knee should be bent and raised to your chest level

Use both hands to grasp behind your leg or calf (avoiding the knee).

Gently straighten your leg as much as possible while maintaining your back level on the ground.

Hold the stretch for 15-30 seconds, and feel a mild pull in the back of your thigh.

Switch legs and repeat the stretch on the opposite side.

***Chair Hamstring Stretch:*** The chair hamstring stretch is a sitting stretch for the muscles at the back of your thighs. Here's how you can accomplish it:

Sit on the edge of a solid chair, feet level on the ground.

Extend one leg out in front of you, heel on the ground, toes pointing up.

Maintain a straight back and bend forward from your hips until you feel a mild stretch at the back of your thigh.

Hold the stretch for 15 to 30 seconds, then switch legs and repeat on the opposite side.

Always take slow breaths and relax into the stretch, avoiding jumping or jerking motions.

This stretch can help increase flexibility in your hamstrings and reduce stiffness, especially if you sit a lot during the day.

***Wall Hamstring Stretch***:

Find an open wall space. Select a clean wall place where you may lie down comfortably with no impediments.

***Lie on your back:*** Position your back flat against the ground. Your legs should be stretched straight out in front of you and parallel to the wall.

***Position yourself:*** Scoot your body up against the wall, getting your buttocks as near to the base as possible. Your legs should be stretched upwards, resting on the wall, with your heels pointed to the ceiling.

Flex your feet by bringing your toes towards your body. This will activate your calf muscles and stretch your hamstrings more efficiently.

***Relax and breathe:*** Take calm, deep breaths as you ease into the stretch. With each breath, work to release any muscle tightness.

Stretch: Hold this posture for 30 seconds to 2 minutes, depending on your flexibility and comfort. You should feel a slight stretch at the back of your thighs and calves.

**Release and repeat:** Slowly drop your legs back to the floor, taking a minute to rest. If desired, you can continue the stretch for another round.

**progressively increase duration:** As your flexibility increases, you may progressively extend the stretch. However, do not push yourself too hard or experience any discomfort when stretching.

**Reclined Hand-to-Big Toe Pose:**

Lie on your back on a yoga mat or a soft surface.

in front of you,Extend both legs straight

Your right knee should be bent and pulled up to your chest level

Wrap a yoga strap or cloth around the arch of your right foot.

Straighten your right leg up to the ceiling, maintaining it as straight as possible.

Hold the strap or towel with both hands, keeping your shoulders relaxed on the mat.

Keep your left leg extended on the mat and press the back of your left thigh down.

Flex your right foot and actively press through the heel.

Gently bring your right leg closer to your body, feeling the stretch at the back of the leg.

breathing deeply and evenly,Hold this position for 30 seconds to 1 minute,

To release, bend your right knee and gently lower your right leg back to the ground.
Repeat the steps with your left leg.

***Dynamic Leg Swings:*** Stand tall and swing one leg forth and backward in a controlled motion, progressively expanding your range of motion.

***Stand Tall:*** Start by standing tall with your feet shoulder-width apart. Use your core muscles and Maintain proper posture

***grip on to Support (Optional):*** To maintain balance, use one hand to grip onto a wall, railing, or other sturdy surface.

***Swing Forward:*** Lift one leg off the ground and swing it forward in a controlled manner. Keep your leg straight but not locked at the knees.

***Swing Backward:*** After swinging your leg forward, let it swing back behind you while maintaining it straight.  A controlled and smooth motion should be used

Repeat on Both Sides.

Swing on one leg for a certain number of repetitions or duration (e.g., 10-15 swings), then switch to the opposite leg.

***Focus on Control and Range of Action:*** Throughout the exercise, maintain control of the swinging action while progressively extending the range of motion as your muscles relax.

***Continue Breathing:*** Remember to breathe rhythmically throughout the activity. Swing your leg forward, then back, inhaling and exhaling.

***Progress Gradually:*** Begin with modest swings and gradually increase the height and intensity as your muscles warm up. Listen to your body and refrain from overstretching.

**Complete Sets:** Perform 2-3 sets of leg swings on each leg, progressively increasing the intensity and range of motion between each set.

**Cool Down:** After finishing the leg swings, do some gentle static stretching or other cool-down exercises to help your muscles relax and stretch.

Dynamic leg swings in a controlled manner to avoid injury and optimize their usefulness as a warm-up activity. If you feel any pain or discomfort, stop immediately and check with a fitness specialist.

Incorporate these hamstring stretches into your morning flexibility practice to enhance your range of motion, relieve muscular tension, and avoid injuries.

**Standing Quadriceps Stretch:** Stand tall, using a support for balance if necessary.

 bring your foot towards your glutes by Bending one knee

Grab your ankle with the appropriate hand and gradually draw it towards your buttocks until you feel a stretch at the front of your thigh.

Hold for 15-30 seconds then swap sides.

***Seated Quadriceps Stretch:***with your legs outstretched in front of you,sit on the floor.
Bend one knee and bring the foot near your buttocks. Hold the ankle and slowly draw it towards you, keeping your spine straight. Hold for 15-30 seconds then swap sides.

***Standing Thigh Stretch:*** Hold one foot behind you with the corresponding hand. Gently move your foot towards your buttocks, keeping your knees tight. Hold for 15-30 seconds then swap sides.

***Lying Quadriceps Stretch:*** Lie on your side, legs piled on top of one another. Bend your top knee and grip your ankle with the top hand. Gently move your ankle towards your buttocks until you feel a stretch in your front thigh. Hold for 15-30 seconds then swap sides.

***Wall Quadriceps Stretch:*** Stand facing a wall with one hand on it for support. Bend one knee and elevate your foot to your buttocks. Press your foot on the wall and feel the stretch in your quadriceps.

Hold for 15-30 seconds then swap sides. Include these exercises in your morning flexibility regimen to increase mobility and prevent muscular stiffness.

Do each stretch slowly and softly, never pushing your body into an uncomfortable position. Stretching should be pleasurable and revitalizing, not unpleasant. Begin your day correctly with these vital quad and thigh stretches!

## *Calf and Achilles Stretching*

When it comes to morning flexibility routines, calf and Achilles stretching is critical for avoiding injury and increasing general mobility. Here is a thorough tutorial geared specifically for you:

***Begin slowly:*** Begin your daily flexibility exercise with a mild warm-up to prepare your muscles for stretching. This might involve mild running, jumping jacks, and dynamic leg swings.

***Calf Stretch:*** Stand facing a wall, one foot in front of the other, toes pointed forward. Keep your rear leg straight and your heel pressed into the ground. Lean forward until you feel a stretch in your calves. Hold for 20-30 seconds and then swap legs.

***Achilles Stretch:*** Sit on the ground with your legs out in front of you. Loop a towel or resistance band over the ball of one foot and gradually pull it towards you, keeping your knee straight. You should feel a stretch at the rear of your leg and Achilles tendon. Hold for 20-30 seconds and then swap legs.

***Standing Calf Stretch:*** Face a wall and place both hands on it at shoulder height. Step one foot back and drive your heel into the ground, keeping your rear leg straight. Lean forward gently till you feel a stretch in your calves. Hold for 20-30 seconds and then swap legs.

***Seated Calf Stretch:*** Sit on the ground with one leg bent and the other stretched straight ahead of you. Wrap a towel or resistance band around the ball of your outstretched foot, then gradually draw it towards you.
A stretch should be felt in your calves.

Hold for 20-30 seconds and then swap legs.

Repeat and Hold.

Stretch each leg 2-3 times, holding for 20-30 seconds each time.

***Listen to Your Body:*** If you experience any severe pain or discomfort, discontinue the stretch immediately. Stretching should not be uncomfortable.

Including these calf and Achilles stretches in your morning flexibility regimen can enhance your overall mobility and lower your chance of injury during exercises.

### Glute and Piriformis Stretches

### Glute Stretch:

Begin by reclining on your back, with both legs bent.

Cross your left ankle over your right knee to form a figure-four formation.

Pull your right knee to your chest with both hands until you feel a stretch in your left glute.

Hold for 20-30 seconds and then swap sides.

Perform 2-3 sets per side.

***Piriformis Stretch:***

Start in a sitting position with both legs outstretched in front of you.

Rest your left foot flat on the floor after Bend your left knee

Over the left kneeCross your right ankle

Gently lean forward with your back straight until you feel a stretch in your right buttock.

Hold for 20-30 seconds and then swap sides.
Repeat for 2-3 sets per side.

Morning flexibility workouts are essential for getting your body ready for the day ahead. These stretches focus on the glutes and piriformis, which can get tight from extended sitting or physical activity.

Stretching these muscles in the morning increases blood flow, relieves stress, and improves general flexibility.

This can help lower the risk of injury during everyday activities and workouts while also improving posture and range of motion.

Incorporate these stretches into your morning routine by doing them before or after your usual workout, or as a stand-alone practice. Hold each stretch for 20-30 seconds and repeat for 2-3 sets on each side.

 Listen to your body and don't overstretch. If you feel any pain or discomfort, stop stretching and get specific advice from a fitness specialist.

Consistency is essential, so make these stretches a daily practice to reap the advantages of increased flexibility and mobility throughout the day.

### *Stretching Routine for Lower Body*

A complete stretching program is vital for improving morning flexibility and lower body mobility. Begin by focusing on key muscle groups, utilizing dynamic stretches to warm up the body and static stretches to improve flexibility. Here's the detailed plan:

***Warm-up (5 minutes):*** Begin with light exercises, such as jogging or jumping jacks, to stimulate blood flow and prepare your muscles for stretching.

***Dynamic Stretches (10 minutes):*** Use dynamic stretches to move your lower-body joints and muscles. Exercises such as leg swings, hip circles, and walking lunges can help to stimulate and stretch muscles at the same time.

Sit on the floor with one leg stretched straight and the other bent inward to stretch your hamstrings (30 seconds per side). Reach towards your toes while maintaining your back straight. Hold the stretch for 30 seconds and then swap sides.

***Quadriceps Stretch (30 seconds on each side):*** Stand tall and raise one foot toward your glutes, holding the ankle with your hand. Gently move your heel towards your buttocks until you feel a stretch in your front thigh. Hold for 30 seconds then switch sides.

***Calf Stretch (30 seconds on each side):*** Stand facing a wall with your hands on it for support. Step one foot back while maintaining it straight, then press your heel into the ground. Lean forward until you feel a stretch in your calves. switch sides after Holding for 30 seconds

***Hip Flexor Stretch (30 seconds on each side):***
Kneel on one knee with the other foot flat on the ground in front of you. Lean forward slightly while maintaining your back straight until you feel a stretch at the front of your hip. Hold for 30 seconds then switch sides.

***Inner Thigh Stretch (30 seconds on each side):***
Sit on the floor with your feet together and your knees bent out to the sides. Gently squeeze your knees down until you feel a stretch in your inner thighs. Hold for 30 seconds.

***Cooldown (5 minutes):*** To relax your muscles and improve healing, end with moderate static stretches or yoga positions like Child's Pose.

By implementing this stretching technique into your morning workout routine, you'll improve your lower body flexibility, minimize your chance of injury, and increase your general mobility for the day.

# CHAPTER FIVE

## *Core Strengthening and Stability*

To begin, be aware  that your core muscles are essential for stability and general body strength. They include muscles in your lower back, hips, and pelvis, as well as your abs. Strengthening these muscles improves posture, balance, and athletic performance while lowering your chance of injury.

Morning flexibility routines that target the core should begin slowly to awaken your muscles. To warm up, try active stretches like leg swings, arm circles, and torso twists. To develop flexibility and range of motion, use static stretches like the cat-cow stretch, the child's posture, and spinal twists.

Continue with core-specific exercises such as planks, side planks, and bird dogs. These exercises work for many muscular groups at the same time, helping to improve stability and strength. Each exercise should be done correctly, with a neutral spine and your core engaged at all times.

Balance exercises such as single-leg stands or stability ball exercises will help you improve your core stability even further. These motions need your core muscles to work harder to maintain balance, which improves general stability and coordination.

As you gain experience, progressively increase the intensity and duration of your morning flexibility workouts. To increase tension and improve your core muscles, try workouts like Russian twists, weighted crunches, or cable rotations.

The most important thing is to be consistent. To observe major increases in core strength and stability over time, do these morning flexibility routines at least three times per week.

If you are uncomfortable or in pain, alter the workouts or get advice from a fitness specialist. With focus and patience, you may build a solid core that will help you with all of your everyday activities and fitness goals.

# Importance of Core Strength

***Stability and balance:*** Your core muscles, which include the abdominals, obliques, and lower back, work together to keep your spine and pelvis stable. This stability is necessary for maintaining balance throughout a variety of tasks, such as lifting weights, jogging, or just standing erect.

***Injury Prevention:*** A strong core lowers the chance of injury by supporting and protecting your spine and surrounding muscles. It promotes appropriate posture, lowering back strain and the risk of overuse problems.

***Improved Performance:*** Whether you're an athlete or just like physical activity, a strong core improves performance. It promotes more efficient movement patterns, greater power transfer, and higher endurance, all of which contribute to better performance in sports and daily activities.

***Functional Movement:*** Core strength is essential for everyday actions including bending, lifting, twisting, and reaching. Improving your core stability and strength allows you to move more effectively and efficiently in all planes of action.

***Enhanced Flexibility:*** While core strength is frequently linked with stability, it also influences flexibility. A healthy core increases overall flexibility since tight muscles in the core can limit mobility elsewhere. Including morning flexibility movements that target the core can assist improve overall flexibility and mobility, resulting in better posture and a lower chance of injury during the day.

Incorporating core-focused workouts into your morning routine improves core strength while also setting a good tone for the day. Aim for a variety of core-targeting exercises, such as planks, bridges, Russian twists, and leg lifts.

listen to your body and advance slowly to avoid overexertion. With constant effort, you'll get the multiple advantages of a strong core, both in workouts and in everyday life.

## *Core Activation Exercises*

When it comes to early flexibility training, core activation exercises are essential for starting your day with strength and stability. These exercises work the muscles in your abdominal, lower back, and pelvis, allowing you to develop a strong foundation for movement and avoid injury throughout the day.

To begin, include exercises such as plank variations in your morning regimen. Begin with a simple plank, keeping your body in a straight line from head to heels. Hold this position for 30-60 seconds, keeping your hips level and activating your core muscles. Gradually increase the time as you gain strength.

Next, incorporate workouts that work the obliques, such as side planks. Lie on your side with your legs stacked and support yourself up on your forearm, elevating your hips to make a straight line. Hold for 30 seconds on each side, experiencing the heat in your side muscles while maintaining stability.

Incorporate dynamic activities, such as mountain climbers or bird dogs, to test your core stability while simultaneously increasing flexibility. For mountain climbers, begin in a plank posture and alternately bring your knees to your chest in a rapid, controlled action. Aim for 10-15 repetitions per leg.

Similarly, bird dogs require you to start on your hands and knees and then extend one arm and the opposing leg at the same time, all while maintaining your core engaged. Hold for a few seconds before returning to the beginning position and repeat on the opposite side. Aim for 10 to 12 repetitions on each side.

Finish your core activation regimen with movements that work the deep stabilizing muscles, such as dead bugs or hollow body holds. These exercises may appear easy, but they are efficient for strengthening the muscles that support your spine and pelvis.

Incorporating these core activation exercises into your morning flexibility regimen will not only enhance your stability and strength but will also prepare you for a productive and injury-free day. To get the most out of each exercise, keep the appropriate form in mind and activate your core muscles.

# Plank Variations

**Standard Plank:** Begin in a push-up position, but rest your weight on your forearms. Maintain a straight line from head to heels while activating your core and glutes. Hold for 30 seconds to a minute while keeping the appropriate form.

**Side Plank:** Lie on your side, elbows just behind your shoulders and legs stacked. Lift your hips until your body is in a straight line from head to heels. Engage your core and hold for 30 seconds to 1 minute on each side. This version addresses the obliques and enhances lateral stability.

**Reverse Plank:** Sit on the floor, legs outstretched in front of you, hands behind your hips. Lift your hips towards the ceiling to form a straight line from head to heels. Hold your core for 30 seconds to a minute. This variant stretches the shoulders, chest, and abdominals while strengthening the posterior chain.

***Plank with Leg Lift:*** Start with the basic plank position. Lift one leg off the ground and maintain your hips level. Hold for a few seconds and then swap legs. This version tests your core stability and increases hip mobility.

***Plank with Arm Raise:*** Begin in the regular plank posture. Lift one arm from the ground and stretch it straight in front of you. Hold for a few seconds, then drop your arm and swap sides. This variant improves shoulder stability while strengthening the core.

Including these plank variants in your morning, flexibility exercise will improve core strength, stability, and general flexibility.

 Aim to hold each variation for 30 seconds to a minute, progressively increasing the length as you improve. Remember to maintain appropriate form and breathing during each exercise to maximize efficiency and avoid injury.

# *Pilates-based exercises*

Pilates focuses on exercising your core muscles, which improves stability and balance while also increasing flexibility by supporting your spine and pelvis.

***Full Body Engagement:*** Pilates movements engage your complete body, targeting muscles that may be missed in typical workouts. This thorough strategy guarantees that you are striving to improve flexibility in all muscle groups.

Pilates focuses on controlled movements with good alignment and form. This not only decreases the chance of injury but also allows you to concentrate on each muscle area, resulting in maximum flexibility increases.

***Dynamic Stretching:*** Many Pilates exercises include dynamic stretching, which includes moving through a range of motion to increase flexibility and mobility. These motions are especially useful for strengthening flexibility in the morning, when your muscles may be tight after sleep.

***Breath Work:*** Pilates emphasizes synchronized breathing and movement, which helps to oxygenate your muscles and allows for deeper stretching. Proper breathing practices encourage relaxation, which leads to increased flexibility.

***Progressive Overload:*** Pilates takes a gradual approach to building flexibility, enabling you to challenge yourself as you gain flexibility. This allows for continued development throughout time.

Pilates promotes a strong mind-body connection, which allows you to become more aware of your body's limitations and possibilities. This understanding enables you to adjust your workouts to target the areas where you require the most flexibility.

Incorporating Pilates-based exercises into your morning flexibility practice will help you start the day feeling energized, renewed, and ready to face whatever obstacles may arise. Whether you're a novice or an experienced practitioner, Pilates is a diverse and effective approach to enhancing your flexibility and general fitness.

# Yoga Poses for Core Strength

To successfully strengthen your core with yoga postures during your morning flexibility training, start with a sequence that targets various muscular groups. Begin in Plank Pose, positioning your wrists behind your shoulders and working your core muscles to maintain a straight line. Hold for 30-60 seconds, focusing on keeping perfect form and deep breathing.

Transition to Side Plank. Pose on each side, raising your hips and raising your upper arm to the ceiling while maintaining your core engaged. Hold for 30 seconds on each side to strengthen your obliques and increase stability.

Next, sit in Boat Pose with your knees bent and feet flat on the floor, then lean back slightly and lift your feet off the ground, balancing on your sit bones. Extend your arms parallel to the floor and hold for 30 seconds, using your core to stay balanced.

Continue with Dolphin Plank Pose, beginning in Dolphin Pose (forearms on the ground, hips elevated) and transferring your weight forward to position your shoulders over your elbows. Engage your core and hold for 30-60 seconds to strengthen the whole core, including your shoulders and upper back.

Continue your sequence with Forearm Plank Pose, which is identical to Plank Pose except that your forearms are on the ground and your elbows are precisely behind your shoulders. Hold for 30-60 seconds, keeping a straight line from your head to your heels and working your core muscles.

Finish your core-strengthening workout with Bridge Pose, which involves lying on your back with knees bent and feet hip-width apart. Lift your hips towards the sky by pressing through your feet, utilizing your glutes and core muscles. Hold for 30 seconds to stretch and strengthen the core and lower back muscles.

Incorporating these yoga postures into your daily flexibility practice will help you not only strengthen your core but also improve your overall balance. Remember to breathe deeply and listen to your body, changing positions as needed to match your flexibility and strength.

# Core Strengthening Routine

To start your morning flexibility workout, focus on dynamic stretching techniques that stimulate your core muscles. Begin with a series of torso twists, side bends, and trunk rotations to warm up your spine and abdominal muscles. These moves will improve blood flow to your core and prepare your body for more strenuous workouts.

Next, include activities that are particularly meant to develop your core muscles. Planks are particularly helpful for this purpose since they work many muscle groups, including the abdominals, obliques, and lower back. Begin with a standard plank posture and hold it for 30 seconds to a minute, gradually increasing the duration as your strength improves.

After planks, try activities that work your lower abdominals, such as leg lifts or reverse crunches. These exercises assist to tighten and tone your lower abdominal muscles, which is essential for general core stability and balance.

Incorporate exercises that need core stability, such as bird dogs or mountain climbers. These exercises not only develop your core muscles but also enhance your balance and coordination, all of which are necessary for daily tasks and sports performance.

Finish your core strengthening practice with a series of stretches to increase flexibility and avoid muscular stiffness. Stretch the muscles that surround your core, such as your hips, hamstrings, and lower back. Hold each stretch for 20-30 seconds, inhaling deeply and trying to relax into the stretch.

Consistency is essential when it comes to core strengthening and flexibility exercises. Aim to execute this exercise at least three times each week, progressively increasing the intensity and length as you advance.

# CHAPTER SIX

## *Cool-down and Relaxation*

After your morning flexibility training, set aside time for a cool-down and relaxation period to maximize the effects and support recovery.

First, participate in a cool-down session to gradually reduce your heart rate and exercise intensity. This prevents blood from accumulating in your extremities, lowering the risk of dizziness or fainting. Begin with 5-10 minutes of low-intensity workouts, such as walking or light jogging.

After that, do static stretching, concentrating on the muscle regions you worked on throughout your workout. Hold each stretch for 15-30 seconds, attempting to release tension and increase flexibility.

Next, enter the relaxation phase to soothe your mind and body. Lie down in a comfortable posture and practice deep breathing exercises by inhaling deeply through your nose and gently expelling through your mouth. This reduces stress hormones and promotes a sense of tranquility.

Incorporate mindfulness methods like progressive muscle relaxation, in which you contract and then relax each muscle group progressively, beginning with your toes and working your way up to your head. Spend 5-10 minutes in this condition, allowing yourself to completely relax and refuel.

Consider integrating yoga or meditation into your post-workout regimen. These techniques not only improve flexibility and mobility but also promote mental clarity and emotional well-being.

Choose positions or practices that help you relax and relieve tension, such as child's pose, corpse pose, or guided meditation. Allow yourself to be present in the moment, letting go of any stress or fears.

After your morning flexibility training, set aside time for a cool-down and relaxation period to promote healing, reduce muscular pain, and improve general well-being. By implementing these activities into your daily routine, you will not only increase your physical performance but also foster a stronger connection between your mind and body.

## *Importance of Cooling Down*

Okay, let's talk about the necessity of a cool-down following your morning flexibility workouts. First and foremost, cooling down is essential because it allows your body to gently shift from intensive physical activity to rest.

***Here's why it is so important:***

***Reduced Risk of Damage:*** After straining your body throughout your morning flexibility program, abruptly stopping might cause muscular discomfort and damage. A thorough cool-down helps your heart rate to gradually drop, preventing blood from accumulating in your muscles, which can lead to cramping and disorientation.

Stretching when cooling down helps to maintain and enhance flexibility. This is especially crucial after a flexibility workout since it helps your muscles to stretch and relax, lowering the likelihood of stiffness later in the day.

***Promotes Recovery:*** A cool-down technique helps to remove metabolic waste products, such as lactic acid, from your muscles. This reduces muscular discomfort and speeds up the recuperation process, allowing you to return to your regular activities sooner.

***Mental Relaxation:*** Cooling down is not only good for your body but also for your mind. It gives a period of peace and relaxation following the intensity of your workout, which aids in stress reduction and promotes overall well-being.

***Long-term Benefits:*** Including a cool-down in your morning flexibility activities can lead to greater athletic performance, better posture, and a lower chance of chronic injuries.

To properly cool down after your morning flexibility program, spend 5-10 minutes doing mild stretching exercises that target the muscles you used throughout your workout. Focus on deep, regulated breathing to help your body relax even more. Alter the intensity of your cool-down according to how you feel. Making cool-downs a regular component of your regimen will improve your flexibility while also promoting general health and well-being.

# *Static Stretching*

When including static stretching in your morning flexibility workouts, it's critical to understand its purpose and execution for the best results.

Static stretching is when you hold a stretch in a comfortable position for an extended amount of time, usually 15-60 seconds. Its primary purpose is to improve flexibility and range of motion by lengthening the muscles and connective tissues.

Before beginning your morning routine, make sure your muscles are warm to avoid damage. Begin with a short warm-up, such as running in place or performing arm circles, to stimulate blood flow and prepare your body for stretching.

Static stretches should target key muscular groups such as the hamstrings, quadriceps, calves, chest, back, and shoulders. Hold each stretch for at least 15-30 seconds, breathing deeply and at a consistent rhythm.

Avoid jumping or jerking motions when static stretching, since they can strain muscles and cause damage. Instead, relax into each stretch until you feel a slight tug, then hold it without pushing beyond your comfort zone.

Include a range of static stretches in your morning routine to target different muscle groups and increase overall flexibility. Experiment with various stretches to see what works best for your body and your requirements.

By including static stretching in your morning flexibility workouts, you may increase your total range of motion, lower your risk of injury, and perform better in other physical activities throughout the day.

## *Deep Breathing Techniques*

Incorporating deep breathing methods into your morning flexibility workout program can dramatically improve its effectiveness. Deep breathing exercises assist to relax your muscles, enhance oxygen flow, and promote flexibility, establishing a good tone for the day ahead.

Begin your morning flexibility workout by locating a quiet, comfortable place to sit or stand straight with proper posture. Close your eyes and start with several rounds of deep diaphragmatic breathing. Inhale deeply through your nose, allowing your abdomen to expand completely.

Feel the breath enter your lungs and expand your chest and ribs. Exhale gently and thoroughly through your lips, squeezing your abdomen to release all of the air.

After you've established a stable rhythm, combine vigorous stretching motions with your breath. As you inhale, gently stretch or reach towards the sky, stretching your spine and activating your muscles. As you exhale, relax the stretch somewhat and sink deeper into the exercise, letting your breath guide you.

Another helpful method is to combine deep breathing and gradual muscular relaxation. As you inhale, tension certain muscular groups in your body, such as your shoulders or legs.

Hold the tension for a moment, then fully exhale as you release the muscles, allowing them to relax entirely. Repeat this practice with different muscle groups throughout your body to progressively improve flexibility and reduce tension.

To improve your morning flexibility routine even more, try mindful breathing methods like alternate nostril breathing or box breathing. These techniques serve to relax the mind, reduce tension, and enhance attention, allowing you to immerse yourself in your workout.

# *Mindfulness meditation*

Mindfulness meditation is an effective technique that may significantly improve your morning flexibility training. Mindfulness meditation trains your mind to be present and aware of sensations, thoughts, and emotions as they emerge, without judgment. This increased awareness extends to your body, allowing you to focus more thoroughly on its signals and motions throughout your flexibility practice.

Start your mindfulness meditation by locating a quiet, comfortable place to sit or lie down. Close your eyes and take a few deep breaths to relax and release tension in your body. As you continue to breathe, draw your attention to the present now, concentrating on the sensations of your breath as it enters and exits your body.

Maintain a sense of focus and awareness as you begin your flexibility training. Pay attention to how your body moves and stretches with each exercise. Identify any places of tightness or discomfort and treat them with gentleness and compassion. Instead of pushing yourself to the limit, be curious and open to exploring your range of motion. Throughout your training, return your focus to your breath whenever your mind wanders. This will help you stay grounded and connected to the present moment, increasing the efficiency of your flexibility exercises.

After you finish your workout, take a few seconds to reflect on how you feel emotionally and physically. Observe any changes or improvements in your flexibility, as well as any changes in your attitude or thinking.

By including mindfulness meditation in your daily flexibility regimen, you may foster a stronger bond between your mind and body, resulting in improved overall health and well-being.

# Relaxation poses

When introducing relaxation poses into your morning flexibility workout program, it's critical to understand their function and how they help your body. Relaxation postures, also known as restorative poses, assist to relieve tension, promote relaxation, and increase flexibility.

***Child's Pose (Balasana):*** Beggin on your hands and knees, then sit back on your heels and extend your arms forward. This posture gently stretches your hips, thighs, and lower back, helping you relax and relieve tension.

***Corpse Pose (Savasana):*** Lie flat on your back, arms at your sides, palms up. Concentrate on deep, rhythmical breathing afternoon closing your eyes. Savasana lets your body completely rest, lowering tension and increasing mental clarity.

***Seated Forward Bend (Paschimottanasana):*** Sit on the floor, legs outstretched in front of you.

Hinge your hips and fold forward, reaching for your feet or shins. This posture stretches the spine, hamstrings, and shoulders, providing relaxation and flexibility.

***Reclining Bound Angle Pose (Supta Baddha Konasana):*** Lie on your back with the soles of your feet touching, allowing your knees to fall wide to the sides. This position softly stretches the inner thighs and groin while relaxing and expanding the hips.

***Legs-Up-the-Wall Pose (Viparita Karani):*** Sit near a wall and lie on your back, stretching your legs up it. Relax your arms at your sides and focus on deep breathing. This position improves circulation, reduces leg strain, and generates a state of relaxation.

Adding these relaxation poses into your morning flexibility practice to loosen up tight muscles, relieve tension, and prepare your mind and body for the day. Remember to hold each posture for at least 1-3 minutes, focusing on deep breathing and letting yourself completely relax. With constant practice, you will notice increased flexibility, lower stress levels, and a better sense of general well-being.

# *Tips for Improved Sleep*

To improve your sleep quality, implement these suggestions into your routine:

***Create a regular sleep schedule:*** Go to bed and wake up at the same time every day, including weekends. your body's internal clock is maintained

Create a calm nighttime ritual. Relax before bedtime by reading, having a warm bath, or practicing relaxation techniques like deep breathing or meditation.

Avoid engaging in stimulating activities such as watching television or using technological gadgets.

Make your sleeping environment favorable to slumber. Ensure that your bedroom is cold, dark, and quiet.

Invest in a comfy mattress and pillows, and use white noise machines or earplugs to drown out any distracting noises.

***Limit your screen time before bedtime:*** Blue light from screens can interfere with your body's generation of melatonin, a hormone that governs sleep. Avoid using electronic gadgets at least an hour before bedtime, or put blue light filters on them.

Limit your caffeine intake, particularly in the afternoon and evening, since it can interfere with your ability to fall asleep. Instead, choose decaffeinated or herbal teas.

***Stay active during the day:*** Regular physical exercise, such as morning flexibility workouts, might help you sleep better. Avoid strenuous activity close to bedtime, since it might energize you and make it difficult to fall asleep.

Monitor your diet: Avoid large meals, spicy foods, and excessive drinks near bedtime, since these might cause discomfort and interrupt your sleep. If you're hungry before bedtime, go for light foods.

***Manage stress:*** Use stress-reduction practices like mindfulness, yoga, or journaling to help you relax and prepare for sleep.

# CHAPTER SEVEN

## Nutrition and Recovery

When it comes to early flexibility training, diet, and recuperation are critical for maximizing performance and outcomes.

**Nutrition:**

**Pre-exercise:** About 1-2 hours before your workout, fuel your body with a well-balanced breakfast or snack high in carbs and moderate in protein. This offers energy to your muscles and helps to prevent weariness.

**Hydration:** Drink water first thing in the morning to help your body rehydrate after sleeping. Drink plenty of water when working out to keep hydrated and perform at your best.

**Post-exercise:** Within 30 minutes after finishing your workout, refuel with a combination of protein and carbs to aid muscle repair and replace glycogen reserves. This might include a protein smoothie, Greek yogurt with fruit, or a turkey sandwich on whole-grain bread.

***Recovery:***

***Cool down:*** After your morning flexibility workout, spend 5-10 minutes doing mild stretching movements to minimize muscle soreness and increase flexibility.

***Rest:*** Get enough sleep every night so your body can mend and recuperate from your exercises. A decent sleep of 7-9 hours should be aimed at

***Active recuperation:*** On rest days, participate in low-intensity activities like walking, yoga, or swimming to stimulate blood flow and healing without overworking your muscles. In addition to post-workout nutrition, eat a well-balanced diet rich in fruits, vegetables, lean proteins, and healthy fats to promote overall recovery and performance.

Prioritizing a healthy diet and recovery techniques can improve the efficacy of your morning flexibility training, lower the chance of injury, and help you reach your fitness objectives more effectively.

## *Importance of Nutrition for Flexibility*

Nutrition is essential for improving flexibility, particularly during early workouts. This is a thorough breakdown:

***Pre-workout Fuel:*** Before your morning flexibility practice, be sure to have a healthy meal or snack. Choose carbs for energy, such as whole grains or fruits, together with protein to assist muscle repair and development, such as yogurt or nuts. This combination gives prolonged energy and prepares your muscles for exercise.

***Hydration:*** Hydration is essential for flexibility. When you wake up, drink water to restore the fluids you lost while sleeping. Aim for constant hydration throughout the day, particularly before and during exercise. Proper hydration keeps your muscles supple and lowers the chance of cramping or stiffness.

*Electrolyte Balance:* Incorporate electrolytes into your morning routine, whether from natural sources such as coconut water or electrolyte-enhanced beverages. Electrolytes aid in maintaining fluid balance and muscular function, which is essential for obtaining maximum flexibility.

*Post-workout Recovery:* After your morning flexibility training, replenish with a good lunch that contains both protein and carbs. This improves muscle repair, lowers pain, and increases flexibility improvements over time. Eggs, lean meats, and healthful grains are great options.

*Anti-inflammatory Foods:* Consume foods with anti-inflammatory characteristics to prevent post-workout inflammation, which can limit flexibility. Incorporate fruits like berries, leafy greens, and omega-3 fatty acids from salmon or flaxseeds into your daily diet.

Consistency is crucial. Make healthy eating a regular habit, not just on activity days. A well-balanced diet promotes general health and helps you keep flexibility throughout time.

***Supplementation:*** To improve joint health and flexibility, consider taking collagen peptides or fish oil. Prioritize whole foods as the basis of your diet. Prioritizing nutrition before, during, and after morning flexibility training is critical for improving performance, lowering injury risk, and meeting long-term flexibility objectives.

By providing your body with the proper nutrients, you may improve your flexibility and general well-being.

# *Hydration Tips*

Hydration is essential for the most effective early flexibility training. Here are some thorough recommendations to help you stay hydrated and perform at your peak:

***Pre-hydration:*** Begin hydrating the night before. Drink 16-20 ounces of water before bed to boost hydration levels in the morning. This prepares your body for the workout ahead.

***Morning Hydration Routine:*** When you wake up, make hydration a priority. Aim to drink another 8-16 ounces of water immediately. This restores fluids lost during sleeping and boosts your metabolism.

***Electrolyte Balance:*** Hydration is more than simply water; electrolytes play an important role. To maintain optimum balance, consume electrolyte-rich meals and beverages such as coconut water, sports drinks, or electrolyte pills.

***Consistent Intake:*** Drink water steadily throughout the day. To avoid dehydration, drink at least 8-10 glasses (64-80 ounces) spaced out evenly. Carry a reusable water bottle as a reminder.

***Monitor Urine Color:*** Use urine color as a hydration indicator. Aim for pale yellow to clear urine, which indicates proper hydration. Dark yellow or amber-colored urine indicates dehydration and necessitates prompt fluid intake.

***Hydrate While Exercising:*** Drink water throughout your morning flexibility workout. Even if you don't feel thirsty as you might after strenuous activity, your body loses fluids through perspiration and respiration.

***Post-Workout Rehydration:*** After your workout, stay hydrated to replenish fluids lost during activity. Aim for another 8-16 ounces of water within 30 minutes to maximize recovery and avoid dehydration.

Listen to Your Body: Everyone has different hydration needs, so pay attention to your body's indications. Thirst is an obvious indication of dehydration, therefore do not disregard it. Adjust your hydration intake according to temperature, humidity, and workout intensity.

Following these complete hydration suggestions can help you achieve optimal fluid balance for your morning flexibility workouts, boosting performance, recovery, and general well-being. Stay hydrated, and flexible, and achieve your exercise objectives!

# *Post-workout nutrition*

Post-exercise nutrition is essential for refilling your body's energy stores, mending muscle tissue, and encouraging recovery after a morning flexibility session. Within 30 minutes to an hour following your activity, strive to eat a balanced supper or snack rich in carbs and protein.

Carbohydrates are vital for refilling glycogen stores that have been exhausted during exercise, allowing your muscles to recuperate and expand. Choose complex carbs such as whole grains, fruits, and vegetables, which give long-term energy and critical nutrients.

Protein is essential for muscle repair and development. Aim for 20-30 grams of high-quality protein each day, which can come from lean meats, poultry, fish, eggs, dairy products, or plant-based choices like tofu or lentils. Consuming protein after a workout increases muscle protein synthesis, which aids in recovery and adaptation to your flexibility practice.

Incorporating a small quantity of healthy fats into your post-workout meal can improve nutrient absorption and provide a consistent source of energy. Incorporate sources such as nuts, seeds, avocados, and olive oil.

Hydration is crucial after an exercise. Drinking water or electrolyte-rich drinks helps to replenish fluids lost via sweating. Drink enough to replenish lost fluids and stay hydrated throughout the day.

If you're short on time or don't feel hungry after your workout, a protein shake or smoothie is an easy alternative. Combine protein powder, fruits, and a source of healthy fats to make a fast and nutritious post-workout snack.

The key to successful post-workout nutrition is timing and balance. To boost recovery and maximize the advantages of your morning flexibility workout, eat a breakfast or snack high in carbs, protein, and healthy fats within an hour of finishing it.

## *Floods to Support Flexibility*

When it comes to promoting flexibility, your food is critical in delivering the nutrients required for your muscles and joints to remain supple and nimble, especially during morning flexibility exercises. Here's a full list of things to include in your diet to help your flexibility regimen:

Include foods high in omega-3 fatty acids, such as salmon, walnuts, chia seeds, and flaxseeds. These fats assist in decreasing inflammation in your joints and promote flexibility.

***Leafy Greens:*** Fill up on spinach, kale, and collard greens. They include vitamins, minerals, and antioxidants that promote joint health and flexibility.

***Protein:*** Make sure you are receiving enough protein from foods like lean meats, tofu, tempeh, and legumes. Protein is required for muscle repair and development, which is critical for maintaining flexibility.

*Citrus Fruits:* Add oranges, lemons, and grapefruits to your diet. They are high in vitamin C, which promotes collagen formation and helps keep your tendons and ligaments flexible.

*Whole Grains:* Opt for whole grains like quinoa, brown rice, and oats over processed grains. Whole grains give continuous energy throughout exercises and contain minerals such as magnesium, which helps relax muscles and promote flexibility.

Turmeric can be added to food or consumed as a tea. Turmeric includes curcumin, an anti-inflammatory substance that can help decrease stiffness and increase flexibility.

*Water:* Stay hydrated all day, especially before and after your morning flexibility workouts. Proper hydration keeps your joints lubricated and prevents cramping, increasing overall flexibility.

By including these items in your diet, you will offer your body the nutrients it requires to maintain flexibility, making your morning workouts more effective and pleasurable. To optimize your flexibility journey, eat a well-balanced diet and pay attention to your body's suggestions.

## *Rest and Recovery Strategies*

Rest and recuperation tactics are essential for optimizing your exercise regimen, especially if you include early flexibility training. Here's a detailed guide on maximizing your rest and recovery:

***Prioritize Sleep:*** Aim for 7-9 hours of good sleep every night to help your body repair and rebuild tissue. Consistent, restful sleep is critical to total healing.

***Nutrition:*** Provide your body with a well-balanced diet high in lean proteins, complex carbs, healthy fats, vitamins, and minerals. Proper eating promotes muscle regeneration and restores energy storage.

Hydration: Stay hydrated throughout the day, particularly after exercise. Water helps to wash out toxins, maintains body temperature, and promotes cellular activity, all of which contribute to healing.

*Active Recovery:* On rest days, incorporate mild exercises such as walking, swimming, or yoga to increase blood flow and release muscles. Active recovery can help improve flexibility and muscular discomfort.

Dynamic stretches should be performed before your morning flexibility training to warm up your muscles and promote blood flow. Static stretching after an exercise can help increase flexibility and minimize the chance of injury.

*Foam rolling:* Use a foam roller to relieve muscular tension. Roll carefully over the target regions, giving soft pressure to relieve knots and enhance mobility.

*Massage Therapy:* Schedule frequent massages to relieve muscle tension, increase circulation, and promote general relaxation. Professional massages can help you recover and avoid overuse injuries.

**Rest Days:** Add rest days to your weekly schedule to allow your body to properly recuperate. Pay attention to your body's signals and adapt your workout level properly to avoid burnout and injury.

**Sleep Hygiene:** Create a nightly routine and a pleasant sleep environment to encourage peaceful sleep. To increase sleep quality, limit your screen time and stimulant exposure before bedtime.

Mindfulness and Stress Management: Use relaxation techniques like meditation, deep breathing, or mild yoga to reduce stress and enhance healing. High-stress levels might impede physical recovery and performance.

Implementing these rest and recovery tactics can help you improve the efficacy of your morning flexibility workouts, increase muscle recovery, avoid injury, and optimize your overall fitness journey. Remember to listen to your body and

adapt your regimen as needed to attain the
greatest results.

# Balancing Workouts and Rest Days

Balancing exercises and rest days is critical for optimizing your fitness journey, especially if you include early flexibility training. Here's a complete guide geared to your requirements:

***Understanding the Importance of Rest Days:*** Rest days are necessary for your muscles to heal and mend. Overtraining can cause weariness, lower performance, and an increased chance of injury. Rest days allow your body time to adjust to the stress of exercise.

***Workout Frequency:*** Aim for flexible workouts in the morning on most days, but don't overdo them. Three to five times a week is an excellent beginning point. To prevent burnout, alternate between intensive and gentle workouts.

Listen to your body. Pay attention to how your body feels. If you're continuously tired or have persistent muscular discomfort, it might be an indication that you need more rest. Adjust your workout program appropriately.

***Workout range:*** To avoid boredom and promote healthy muscular growth, do a range of flexibility exercises. Include stretching, yoga, and mobility exercises in your program. This diversification not only promotes flexibility but also lowers the likelihood of overuse problems.

***Active Recovery:*** On rest days, participate in physical activities such as walking, swimming, or mild yoga. These activities increase blood flow, enhance muscle healing, and reduce discomfort.

***Quality Sleep:*** Make sure you are receiving enough sleep since it is critical for muscle restoration and general recovery. Aim for 7-9 hours of excellent sleep every night to help you achieve your fitness objectives.

***Diet and Hydration:*** Proper diet and hydration are critical to recovery. Fuel your body with nutrient-dense meals and remain hydrated throughout the day to improve your performance and recovery.

***Periodization:*** Use periodization in your training regimen by alternating between high-intensity exercises and recuperation periods. This systematic method minimizes plateaus and lowers the likelihood of overtraining.

By adhering to these rules, you may properly balance your morning flexibility sessions with rest days, maximizing your development while reducing the danger of burnout and injury.

Note that perseverance and patience are essential in your fitness quest.

# CONCLUSION

Morning flexibility workouts have several benefits that go beyond physical flexibility. Individuals may improve their general health and performance throughout the day by taking a complete strategy that includes stretching, mobility exercises, and mindful movement.

For starters, morning flexibility activities improve joint mobility and alleviate stiffness that has built up over the night. These workouts awaken and prepare the body for the day ahead by integrating dynamic stretches and soft movements, lowering the chance of injury and improving general physical function.

Flexibility exercises enhance posture and alignment, which can help with common concerns like back discomfort and tension headaches. Regular morning flexibility practices can help people develop improved body awareness and healthier movement patterns, resulting in long-term musculoskeletal health.

Morning flexibility workout can provide considerable mental health advantages. The purposeful concentration on breath and movement promotes awareness and presence, which sets a positive tone for the day ahead. This mindful technique can help people better handle stress and improve their general mental clarity and attention.

Additionally, morning flexibility practices allow for self-care and introspection. Taking time each morning to prioritize one's physical and mental well-being establishes a strong goal for the day, encouraging increased self-awareness and self-esteem.

Adding diversity to morning flexibility workouts, such as trying out different yoga types or combining components of Pilates or Tai Chi, can boost their efficiency and keep them from becoming monotonous. This diversity not only challenges the body in novel ways but also keeps the mind active and motivated.

Morning flexibility workouts promote physical health, mental well-being, and emotional resilience, making them an all-around way to start the day. Individuals can get long-term benefits by incorporating them into their daily routine.

Thank you for selecting this book. Your support is really appreciated. Similarly, I am grateful for the purchase of this book. Your input is valuable; please share your ideas in a review. It serves as a reference for future improvements. Enjoy reading and utilizing it!

# *Workout Planner to help track progress*

# Workout Planner to keep Track of progress

|         | EXERCISE | GOAL |
|---------|----------|------|
| MON DAY |          |      |
| TUES DAY |         |      |
| WEDNES DAY |       |      |
| THURS DAY |        |      |
| FRI DAY |          |      |
| SAT DAY |          |      |

| | EXERCISE | GOAL |
|---|---|---|
| MON DAY | | |
| TUES DAY | | |
| WEDNES DAY | | |
| THURS DAY | | |
| FRI DAY | | |
| SAT DAY | | |

| | EXERCISE | GOAL |
|---|---|---|
| MON DAY | | |
| TUES DAY | | |
| WEDNES DAY | | |
| THURS DAY | | |
| FRI DAY | | |
| SAT DAY | | |

# Workout Planner to keep Track of progress

| | EXERCISE | GOAL |
|---|---|---|
| MON DAY | | |
| TUES DAY | | |
| WEDNES DAY | | |
| THURS DAY | | |
| FRI DAY | | |
| SAT DAY | | |

| | EXERCISE | GOAL |
|---|---|---|
| MON DAY | | |
| TUES DAY | | |
| WEDNES DAY | | |
| THURS DAY | | |
| FRI DAY | | |
| SAT DAY | | |

# Workout Planner to keep Track of progress

| | EXERCISE | GOAL |
|---|---|---|
| MONDAY | | |
| TUESDAY | | |
| WEDNESDAY | | |
| THURSDAY | | |
| FRIDAY | | |
| SATDAY | | |